CIALIS

Your Effective Manual on How to Safely and Effectively Use Cialis

MORGAN PRICE

Cialis

Cialis is a drug used to treat erectile dysfunction in men. Erectile dysfunction is a condition that affects sexual performance in men, where the penis does not harden and grow erect when the male is sexually stimulated. This can be a source of problem in the relationship, due to lack of sexual performance. With Cialis, you don't have to worry about this deficiency. It helps retain erection after the penis is caressed, by increasing the flow of blood to the penis.

Cialis is also used to cure men suffering from benign prostatic hyperplasia. This condition is caused by an enlarged prostate; this condition makes it hard for men to urinate. Using Cialis would make the signs and symptoms less serious and reduce the chances of opting for prostate surgery.

The medication is equally used for both men and

women to treat pulmonary arterial hypertension, thereby, enhancing your capacity to exercise. The medication is only available as an oral suspension and tablet. Keep in mind that this medication does not prevent sexually transmitted infections (STIs). To play safe, use condoms while having sex.

Remember to use this drug according to the directives of your doctor. Don't use more or less than the prescribed dose.

Things to Keep in Mind When Using This Medication

Knowing important things about this medication would help you avoid some complications before or while using this drug.

- If you have a history of being allergic to this medication or the ingredients used in making Cialis, inform your doctor to know if it is safe to use the drug. If you have other allergies, do well to inform the doctor.

- The usefulness of this drug is reduced by elderly folks. Also, they are more vulnerable to the side effects of this medication.

- This medication can cause extreme

dizziness. To be on the safe side, don't drive or engage in physical activities that require mental alertness, to avoid endangering yourself, until the effects of the medication are ascertained.

- There has been no proof that this

medication can endanger the infant when used by a breastfeeding mother. Regardless, before using the drug, do well to seek the advice of your doctor.

- Cialis does not prevent sexually transmitted diseases (STIs) when engaging in sexual activities. To be on the safe side, use condoms to avoid sexually transmitted infections.

- Come clean about your medical history when using this drug. If you have liver problems, heart disease, kidney disease, stroke in the past 6 months, stomach ulcer, low blood pressure, high blood pressure, sudden decrease in vision, and other problems, inform your doctor to know if you can use the medication or not.

- The dose or length of time you would use this medication depends on your current health condition, body response to treatment, and other drugs you are using.

Side Effects of Using Cialis

Using Cialis comes with its side effects. Some of the side effects don't require the attention of a doctor, while some require immediate medical attention. If the condition continues for a long time or gives you discomfort, inform your doctor and stop using the medication. Below are the side effects of using Cialis:

- inability to speak
- joint or muscle pain
- losing of heat from the body
- numbness or tingling of the face, hands, or feet

- red skin lesions, usually with a purple center
- red, painful eyes
- red, swollen skin
- redness of the skin
- redness or soreness of the eyes
- scaly skin
- sluggish speech
- sores, ulcers, or white blotches in the mouth or on the lips

- stomach discomfort
- premature cardiac death
- bulging of the feet or lower legs
- Arm, back, or jaw pain
- clouded vision
- chest ache, pain, tightness, or adiposity
- colds
- cold sweats
- bewilderment
- tiredness

- fainting
- faintness or lightheadedness when getting up unawares from a lying or sitting position
- quick or irregular heartbeat
- headache
- hearing failure
- increased erection
- sickness
- anxiety

- discomfort or distress in the arms, jaw, back, or neck
- complication with speaking
- double vision
- fast, unstable, thumping, or racing heartbeat or pulsation
- headache, severe and throbbing

- hives or bruises, itching, skin inflammation
- increased erection
- nausea
- nervousness
- pain or discomfort in the arms, jaw, back, or neck
- battering in the ears
- unhurried or rapid heartbeat

- spontaneous penile erection
- sweating
- uncommon drowsiness or weakness
- puking
- Unbearable or lengthened erection of the penis
- blistering, peeling, or loosening of the skin
- cough
- ruptures in the skin

- decline or shift in vision
- diarrhea.

How to Use Cialis

It is important to know how to use this medication, as it would help you get the best out of this medication. Below are the ways to use Cialis:

- Read the instructions on the leaflet left by the manufacturer. If there is anything you find confusing, ask your doctor for directions on how it works. Don't use more than the prescribed dose, longer than the recommended length of time, or more often than prescribed to avoid complications.

- The dosage prescribed by the doctor has to do with the health condition you are treating, your body's response to drugs, and the other medications you are using.

- The medication can be used with or without food, depending on the instruction of your doctor. Swallow the medication in full, there is no need to split, chew, or break the drug before use.

- Use only the brand of Cialis recommended by your doctor because the functions of the various brands might differ.

- Use the medication for the full length of time prescribed by your doctor to have the best effect.

We Appreciate You For Reading!!!

Printed in Great Britain
by Amazon

37837174R00020